HOW TO MAKE NATURAL ANTI-WRINKLE CREAMS & ANTI-AGING SERUMS

DR MIRIAM KINAI

ISBN: 1492709697

ISBN-13: 978-1492709695

CONTENTS

DR MIRIAM KINAI

1

BASIC ANTI-WRINKLE CREAM

ANTI-WRINKLE CREAM MAKING EQUIPMENT

2 glass bowls

Double boiler

Sieve and cheesecloth

Wide mouthed containers with tight fitting lids

*****

ANTI-WRINKLE CREAM RECIPE INGREDIENTS

1 oz. (30 grams) beeswax

1 oz. (30 grams) virgin coconut oil

3 fl oz. (90 ml) therapeutic vegetable oils like apricot kernel oil and avocado oil

3 fl oz (90 ml) sweet almond oil to make a herb infused oil

1 oz. dry herbs or 2 oz. fresh herbs like calendula, chamomile, lavender

50 drops of essential oils like lavender essential oil

1 teaspoon vitamin E oil (optional natural preservative)

*****

BASIC ANTI-WRINKLE CREAM RECIPE INSTRUCTIONS

1. Place the dry herbs or fresh herbs and 3 oz of sweet almond oil in a glass bowl ensuring that the oil covers the herbs. Simmer them in a double boiler for one hour at around 120 degrees Fahrenheit (49 degrees Celsius). Strain the mixture through a sieve and cheesecloth into a clean bowl.

2. Melt the beeswax, virgin coconut oil and therapeutic vegetable oils in a double boiler while stirring or in the microwave for several 10 second bursts. Remove them from the heat source and let them cool for a few minutes.

3. Add the essential oils drop by drop as you stir until you get your desired scent.

4. Add the vitamin E oil (optional natural preservative).

5. Pour the mixture into a wide mouthed container with a tight fitting lid and store it in a cool, dark place.

Tip

You can use 6 oz. of plain vegetable oils if you do not want to make the herb infused oils. You can also use 6 oz. of herb infused oils to make your anti-wrinkle cream.

* * * * *

2

THERAPEUTIC ANTI-WRINKLE CREAM RECIPES

Normal Skin Recipe

1 oz. (30 grams) beeswax

1 oz. (30 grams) virgin coconut oil

3 fl oz. (90 ml) vegetable oils used on normal skin like jojoba, sweet almond oil, olive oil, sunflower oil, apricot kernel oil and avocado oil.

3 fl oz (90 ml) sweet almond oil to make a herb infused oil

1 oz. dry herbs or 2 oz. fresh herbs used on normal skin like chamomile flowers, lavender flowers, rosemary, arnica, calendula flowers and comfrey.

50 drops of essential oils that can be used on normal skin like clary sage, eucalyptus, geranium, grapefruit, lavender, lemon, lemongrass, Roman chamomile, spearmint, sweet orange, rosemary, peppermint, tea tree and ylang ylang.

1 teaspoon vitamin E oil (optional natural preservative)

Follow the above Basic Anti-Wrinkle Cream Recipe Instructions.

***

Dry Skin Recipe

1 oz. (30 grams) beeswax

1 oz. (30 grams) virgin coconut oil

3 fl oz. (90 ml) therapeutic vegetable oils that are perfect for dry skin like sweet almond oil, sunflower oil, jojoba, avocado oil, apricot kernel, olive, evening primrose, virgin coconut, fractionated coconut oil, calendula oil

3 fl oz (90 ml) sweet almond oil to make a herb infused oil

1 oz. dry herbs or 2 oz. fresh herbs used to manage dry skin like calendula flowers, chamomile flowers, lavender flowers, rosemary leaves, comfrey

50 drops of essential oils used to manage dry skin like lavender, Roman chamomile, ylang ylang

1 teaspoon vitamin E oil (optional natural preservative)

Follow the above Basic Anti-Wrinkle Cream Recipe Instructions.

***

Sensitive Skin Recipe

1 oz. (30 grams) beeswax

1 oz. (30 grams) virgin coconut oil

3 fl oz. (90 ml) therapeutic vegetable oils that are perfect for sensitive skin like apricot kernel oil, sweet almond, avocado oil

3 fl oz (90 ml) sweet almond oil to make a herb infused oil

1 oz. dry herbs or 2 oz. fresh herbs used to manage sensitive skin like calendula flowers, chamomile flowers, lavender flowers

50 drops of essential oils like lavender and Roman chamomile

1 teaspoon vitamin E oil (optional natural preservative)

Follow the above Basic Anti-Wrinkle Cream Recipe Instructions.

***

Oily and Acne Prone Skin Recipe

1 oz. (30 grams) beeswax

1 oz. (30 grams) virgin coconut oil

3 fl oz. (90 ml) therapeutic vegetable oils that are perfect for oily skin like jojoba, sweet almond oil

3 fl oz (90 ml) sweet almond oil to make a herb infused oil

1 oz. dry herbs or 2 oz. fresh herbs used to manage oily skin like turmeric powder, cinnamon powder, lavender flowers, rose petals, lemongrass, witch hazel or dried crushed neem leaves

50 drops of essential oils used to manage oily skin and acne like tea tree, lemon, lavender, sandalwood

1 teaspoon vitamin E oil (optional natural preservative)

Follow the above Basic Anti-Wrinkle Cream Recipe Instructions.

Eczema Prone Skin Recipe

1 oz. (30 grams) beeswax

1 oz. (30 grams) virgin coconut oil

3 fl oz. (90 ml) therapeutic vegetable oils used to manage eczema like evening primrose oil, rose hip oil, cranberry seed oil, calendula, coconut oil, sweet almond oil, borage seed oil and jojoba

3 fl oz (90 ml) sweet almond oil to make a herb infused oil

1 oz. dry herbs or 2 oz. fresh herbs used to manage eczema like calendula flowers, chamomile flowers

50 drops of essential oils used to manage eczema like geranium, lavender, Roman chamomile and rosemary

1 teaspoon vitamin E oil (optional natural preservative)

Follow the above Basic Anti-Wrinkle Cream Recipe Instructions.

***

Psoriasis Prone Skin Recipe

1 oz. (30 grams) beeswax

1 oz. (30 grams) virgin coconut oil

3 fl oz. (90 ml) vegetable oils that manage psoriasis like cranberry seed, borage seed, carrot seed, evening primrose, calendula, jojoba

3 fl oz (90 ml) sweet almond oil to make a herb infused oil

1 oz. dry herbs or 2 oz. fresh herbs used to manage psoriasis like chamomile flowers, calendula, chickweed, comfrey root

50 drops essential oils that treat psoriasis like bergamot, tea tree, rose, lavender, German chamomile, helichrysum, patchouli, sandalwood

1 teaspoon vitamin E oil (optional natural preservative)

Follow the above Basic Anti-Wrinkle Cream Recipe Instructions.

Mature Skin Recipe

1 oz. (30 grams) beeswax

1 oz. (30 grams) virgin coconut oil

3 fl oz. (90 ml) therapeutic vegetable oils that are perfect for mature skin like evening primrose, avocado, apricot kernel, jojoba, sweet almond, olive

3 fl oz (90 ml) sweet almond oil to make a herb infused oil

1 oz. dry herbs or 2 oz. fresh herbs used to manage mature skin like calendula flowers, chamomile flowers, lavender flowers, green tea leaves, rose petals

50 drops of essential oils essential oils used to manage mature skin like rose, geranium, clary sage, lavender

1 teaspoon vitamin E oil (optional natural preservative)

Follow the above Basic Anti-Wrinkle Cream Recipe Instructions.

***

Prematurely Aging Skin Recipe

1 oz. (30 grams) beeswax

1 oz. (30 grams) virgin coconut oil

3 fl oz. (90 ml) therapeutic vegetable oils that are perfect for prematurely aging skin like apricot kernel, carrot, wheat germ, evening primrose, sweet almond oil

3 fl oz (90 ml) sweet almond oil to make a herb infused oil

1 oz. dry herbs or 2 oz. fresh herbs used to manage prematurely aging skin like calendula flowers, chamomile flowers, lavender flowers, green tea leaves, rose petals

50 drops of essential oils used to manage prematurely aging skin like patchouli, clary sage, rose, lavender, geranium

1 teaspoon vitamin E oil (optional natural preservative)

Follow the above Basic Anti-Wrinkle Cream Recipe Instructions.

* * * * *

3

BASIC ANTI-AGING SERUM

ANTI-AGING SERUM MAKING EQUIPMENT

Bottle with a dropper top

*****

ANTI-AGING SERUM RECIPE INGREDIENTS

1 oz. (30 ml) vegetable oil

5 drops essential oil

1 teaspoon vitamin E oil (optional natural preservative with anti-oxidant properties)

*****

ANTI-AGING SERUM RECIPE INSTRUCTIONS

1. Combine all the ingredients in a bottle with a dropper top. Roll the bottle in your palm to mix the ingredients.

* * * * *

4

THERAPEUTIC ANTI-AGING SERUMS

Normal Skin Recipe

1 oz. (30 ml) vegetable oil used on normal skin like jojobo, sweet almond oil, virgin coconut, olive oil, sunflower oil, apricot kernel oil, sweet almond, avocado oil

5 drops essential oil used on normal skin like clary sage, eucalyptus, geranium, grapefruit, lavender, lemon, lemongrass, Roman chamomile, spearmint, sweet orange, rosemary, peppermint, tea tree and ylang ylang

1 teaspoon vitamin E oil

Follow the above Basic Anti-Aging Face Serum Recipe Instructions.

Dry Skin Recipe

1 oz. (30 ml) vegetable oil that are perfect for dry skin like sweet almond oil, sunflower oil, jojoba, avocado oil, apricot kernel, olive, evening primrose, virgin coconut, fractionated coconut oil, calendula oil

5 drops essential oils used to manage dry skin like lavender, Roman chamomile, ylang ylang

1 teaspoon vitamin E oil (optional natural preservative with anti-oxidant properties)

Follow the above Basic Anti-Aging Face Serum Recipe Instructions.

***

Sensitive Skin Recipe

1 oz. (30 ml) vegetable oils that are perfect for sensitive skin like apricot kernel oil, sweet almond, avocado oil

5 drops essential oils used to manage sensitive skin like lavender, Roman chamomile

1 teaspoon vitamin E oil (optional natural preservative with anti-oxidant properties)

Follow the above Basic Anti-Aging Face Serum Recipe Instructions.

***

Oily and Acne Prone Skin Recipe

1 oz. (30 ml) vegetable oils that are perfect for oily skin like jojoba, sweet almond oil

5 drops essential oils used to manage oily skin and acne like tea tree, lemon, lavender, sandalwood

1 teaspoon vitamin E oil (optional natural preservative with anti-oxidant properties)

Follow the above Basic Anti-Aging Face Serum Recipe Instructions.

Eczema Prone Skin Recipe

1 oz. (30 ml) vegetable oils that manage eczema like evening primrose, rose hip, cranberry seed, calendula, sweet almond, borage seed and jojoba

5 drops essential oils used to manage eczema like geranium, lavender, Roman chamomile and rosemary

1 teaspoon vitamin E oil

Follow the above Basic Anti-Aging Face Serum Recipe Instructions.

***

Psoriasis Prone Skin Recipe

1 oz. (30 ml) vegetable oils used to manage psoriasis like cranberry seed oil, borage seed oil, evening primrose oil, calendula, carrot seed oil, jojoba and coconut oil

5 drops essential oils used to manage psoriasis like bergamot, tea tree, lavender, German chamomile, helichrysum, patchouli, rose and sandalwood

1 teaspoon vitamin E oil (optional natural preservative with anti-oxidant properties)

Follow the above Basic Anti-Aging Face Serum Recipe Instructions.

***

Mature Skin Recipe

1 oz. (30 ml) vegetable oils that are perfect for mature skin like evening primrose, avocado, apricot kernel, jojoba, sweet almond, olive

5 drops essential oils used to manage mature skin like rose, geranium, clary sage, lavender essential oils

1 teaspoon vitamin E oil (optional natural preservative with anti-oxidant properties)

Follow the above Basic Anti-Aging Face Serum Recipe Instructions.

Prematurely Aging Skin Recipe

1 oz. (30 ml) vegetable oils that are perfect for prematurely aging skin like apricot kernel, carrot, wheat germ, evening primrose, sweet almond oil

5 drops essential oils used to manage prematurely aging skin like patchouli, clary sage, rose, lavender, geranium

1 teaspoon vitamin E oil (optional natural preservative with anti-oxidant properties)

Follow the above Basic Anti-Aging Face Serum Recipe Instructions.

Follow the above Basic Face Scrub Recipe Instructions.

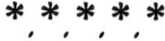

5

VEGETABLE OILS

Choose the vegetable oils you will use for your natural skincare products depending on your skin type and the condition that you want the product to manage.

Sweet Almond Oil

Sweet almond oil contains vitamins A, B, E, minerals and skin nourishing essential fatty acids. It is especially beneficial for normal skin, dry skin, sensitive skin, mature skin and eczema prone skin.

Do not use sweet almond oil if you have nut allergy.

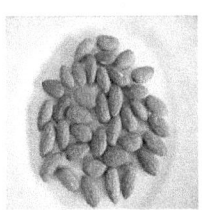

Sunflower Oil

Sunflower oil contains vitamin A, E and skin nourishing essential fatty acids. It is especially beneficial for normal skin and dry skin.

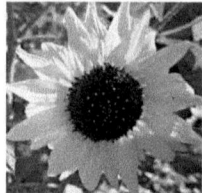

***

Avocado Oil

Avocado oil is rich in skin nourishing nutrients. It is especially beneficial for normal skin, dry skin, sensitive skin, mature skin, eczema prone skin and psoriasis prone skin.

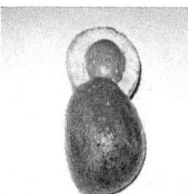

***

Apricot Kernel Oil

Apricot kernel oil contains vitamins A, E, minerals and skin nourishing essential fatty acids. It is especially beneficial for dry skin, sensitive skin, mature skin and prematurely aging skin.

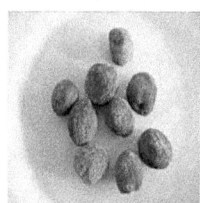

Jojoba

Jojoba is a plant wax which contains vitamin E, proteins, minerals and skin nourishing fatty acids and protective antioxidants. It is especially beneficial for normal skin, mature skin, oily or acne prone skin, eczema prone skin and psoriasis prone skin.

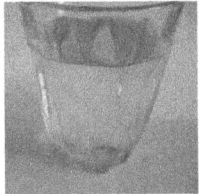

***

Olive Oil

Olive oil contains skin nourishing essential fatty acids and natural sunscreens. It is especially beneficial for dry skin, mature skin and eczema prone skin. It is also conditions nails.

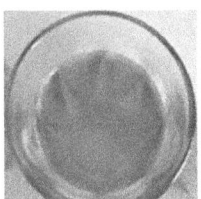

***

Virgin Coconut Oil

Virgin coconut oil contains skin nourishing fatty acids. It is especially beneficial for dry skin. It also conditions nails.

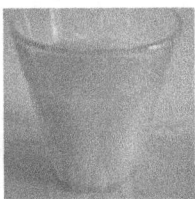

Fractionated Coconut Oil

Fractionated coconut oil is especially beneficial for dry skin and sensitive skin.

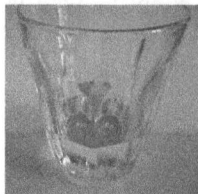

***

Canola Oil

Canola oil is especially beneficial for normal skin, dry skin, sensitive skin and mature skin.

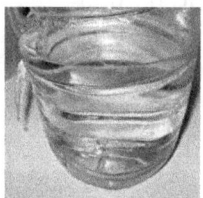

***

Evening Primrose Oil

Evening primrose oil contains skin nourishing essential fatty acids, vitamins and minerals. It is especially beneficial for dry skin, mature skin, eczema prone skin and psoriasis prone skin.

* * * * *

6

ESSENTIAL OILS

Choose the aromatherapy essential oils you will use for your natural skincare products depending on your skin type and the condition that you want the product to manage.

Clary Sage Essential Oil

Clary Sage Essential Oil has an herbaceous scent. It can help relieve stress related tension, reduce irritability and help one relax. It is also used for the management of mature and acne prone skin.

Do not use it during pregnancy or if you are drinking alcohol or driving or if you have endometriosis, ovarian cysts, uterine cysts, breast cancer or you are at high risk for developing breast cancer as it may have an "estrogen-like" effect on the body.

***

Eucalyptus Essential Oil

Eucalyptus essential oil has an invigorating scent. It can help relieve stress related mental tension and mental exhaustion. It is also used in the management of joint aches and pains.

Do not use eucalyptus essential oil if you have epilepsy, high blood pressure or apply it near a baby's nostrils.

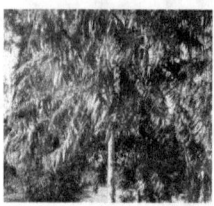

***

Geranium Essential Oil

Geranium Essential Oil has a fresh, minty rose scent. It can help relieve nervous tension and anxiety. It is also used in the management of eczema, cellulite as well as mature skin.

Avoid using it in pregnancy.

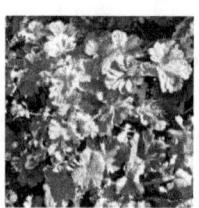

***

Grapefruit Essential Oil

Grapefruit essential oil has a refreshing, bitter-sweet scent. It can help relieve tension and release repressed emotions. It is also used in the management of cellulite.

Lavender Essential Oil

Lavender essential oil has a soothing, floral scent. It can help one relax and relieve stress related tension, sleeplessness, anxiety and depression. It is also used in the management of **acne, eczema and dry skin** conditions.

Do not use lavender essential oil in pregnancy, if you are breastfeeding, on young children as it may cause breast development in young boys and girls. Avoid it if you have low blood pressure as you may feel drowsy after using it.

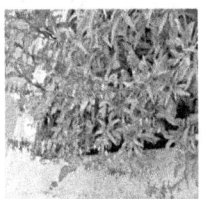

***

Lemon Essential Oil

Lemon essential oil has a clarifying fresh scent. It can help relieve mental tension, alleviate mental fatigue and increase concentration. It is also used in the management of acne and post acne dark skin spots.

Do not use it if skin will be exposed to sunlight or UV rays in the next 12-24 hours. Do not use it if you have low blood pressure or you are allergic to lemons.

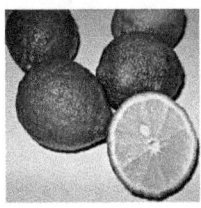

Lemongrass Essential Oil

Lemongrass essential oil has a vitalizing, lemony scent. It can help relieve tension and muscle aches. It is also used in the management of acne.

Do not use it if skin will be exposed to sunlight or UV rays in the next 12-24 hours.

Roman Chamomile Essential Oil

Roman chamomile essential oil has a sweet and fruity scent. It can help relieve stress related tension headaches. It is also used in the management of eczema, psoriasis and dry skin conditions.

Avoid using it in pregnancy and if you are allergic to ragweed.

***

Spearmint Essential Oil

Spearmint essential oil has a gently-energizing minty scent. It can help relieve mental tension and exhaustion. It is also used in the management of nausea.

***

Rose Essential Oil

Rose essential oil has a sweet and floral scent. It has mentally cheering properties and is used to relieve **depression, sorrow and heartache**. It is also useful for mature and prematurely aging skin.

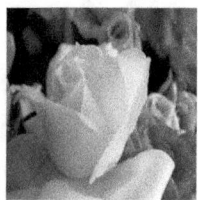

Rosemary Essential Oil

Rosemary Essential Oil has an uplifting and stimulating scent. It can help relieve mental exhaustion and feeling rundown. It is also used in the management of dry skin, eczema, muscle aches and joint pains.

Do not use rosemary essential oil if you are pregnant or have epilepsy or high blood pressure. Avoid using it if you have a fever or you want to sleep and in children under 5 years.

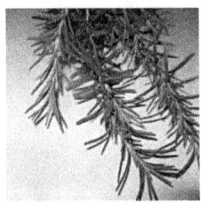

***

Sweet Orange Essential Oil

Sweet orange essential oil has a cheeringly, refreshing scent. It can help mange stress related tension. It is also used in the management of cellulite and common colds.

Do not use it if skin will be exposed to sunlight or UV rays in the next 12-24 hours.

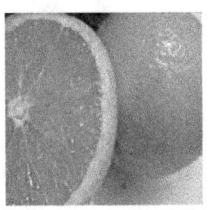

***

Peppermint Essential Oil

Peppermint essential oil has a head-clearing, refreshing scent. It can help relieve tension and fatigue. It is also used to manage flatulence.

Do not use peppermint essential oil in pregnancy, if breastfeeding, on children less than 5 years, if you have epilepsy or irregular heartbeats or cardiac fibrillation or high blood pressure and before using a sun bed or going to hot humid places.

***

Tea Tree Essential Oil

Tea tree essential oil has a purifying almost medicinal scent. It can help relieve tension and fatigue. It is also been used in the management of oily skin, acne and athlete's foot.

***

Ylang Ylang Essential Oil

Ylang ylang essential oil has a fragrantly floral scent. It can help relieve anxiety, tension and help one relax. It is also used as an aphrodisiac and in the management of dry skin conditions.

Do not use ylang ylang essential oil if you have low blood pressure or sensitive, damaged skin.

* * * * *

7

HERBS

Choose the herbs you will use for your natural skincare products depending on your skin type and the condition that you want the product to manage.

Aloe Vera

Aloe vera has anti-inflammatory properties and acts as a soothing balm for inflamed skin. It also stimulates cell regeneration and is vital for healing. Since it contains over 90% water, it is also an excellent moisturizer.

***

Arnica Flowers

Arnica flowers are believed to have anti-inflammatory properties and are used to relieve the pains of sprains, muscle aches and joint pains.

Do not use arnica if you are allergic to it, if pregnant or breastfeeding.

Calendula Flowers

Calendula flowers are used to manage dry, sensitive, mature, prematurely aging and normal skin types.

Calendula flowers also have antioxidant, anti-inflammatory and anti-infective properties. They are therefore also used to help wounds, minor cuts and bruises, small insect bites, first degree burns, mild sunburns and mild skin infections heal faster.

Calendula is also a soothing agent which reduces inflammation and it has been shown to prevent dermatitis or skin inflammation in breast cancer patients receiving radiation treatment.

Do not use calendula if you are allergic to it, allergic to daisy or aster family plants like ragweed and chrysanthemums, if pregnant or breastfeeding or trying to conceive. Avoid calendula preparations if you are taking sedatives, high blood pressure and diabetes medications.

***

Chamomile Flowers

Chamomile flowers are used to manage dry, sensitive, oily, mature, prematurely aging and normal skin types.

Chamomile flowers have anti-inflammatory activity and mild antiseptic properties. They are also soothing to the skin and help in eliminating blackheads by helping open up the pores.

Chamomile flowers also have mentally relaxing properties and are used to relieve anxiety and emotional stress.

Do not use/ avoid chamomile if you are allergic to it, allergic to daisy or aster family plants like ragweed and chrysanthemums, have asthma, if pregnant as it may cause miscarriage, if driving as it may cause drowsiness, if taking alcohol, for at least 2 weeks before surgery or dental procedures as it may cause bleeding.

Do not use/avoid chamomile if you are taking blood thinners like warfarin (coumadin), clopidogrel (plavix) or aspirin as it may cause bleeding, sedatives, high blood pressure and diabetes medications.

Comfrey Leaves

Comfrey leaves are used to manage dry and normal skin types.

Comfrey leaves have anti-inflammatory, skin regenerative and antiseptic properties. They are also used to relieve muscle strains and ligament sprains.

Do not use/ avoid comfrey if you are allergic to it, on broken skin, on children, the elderly, if pregnant or breastfeeding, in liver disease, alcoholism and cancer.

Do not use/ avoid comfrey if you are taking acetaminophen (panadol, tylenol). Do not use/ avoid comfrey if using herbs known to cause liver problems such as kava, valerian, skullcap and pennyroyal.

***

Lavender Flowers

Lavender flowers are used to treat eczema and manage dry, sensitive, mature, prematurely aging, normal, oily and acne prone skin.

Lavender flowers have calming, analgesic, anti-inflammatory and skin regenerative properties. They are also used to manage stress, reduce anxiety and insomnia and relieve muscle and joint aches.

Do not use/ avoid lavender if you are allergic to it, on broken skin, if pregnant or breastfeeding, on young boys as it may cause male breast development. Do not use/ avoid lavender if you are taking sedatives, anti-anxiety medications such as lorazepam and narcotic analgesics such as morphine and oxycodone.

***

Rose Petals

Rose petals are used to manage oily, mature and prematurely aging skin.

Rose petals are also believed to have skin softening properties.

Rosemary Leaves

Rosemary leaves are used to manage dry and normal skin.

Rosemary leaves have antioxidant and antimicrobial properties. They are mentally stimulating and are used to reduce feelings of sadness or depression, increase mental concentration and relieve muscle pains and joint aches.

Do not use/ avoid rosemary if you are allergic to it, are breastfeeding or pregnant as it may cause miscarriages, are under 18 years old, have high blood pressure, peptic ulcers, ulcerative colitis or Crohn's disease. Do not use/avoid rosemary if you are taking blood thinners such as warfarin (coumadin), clopidogrel (plavix) or aspirin as it may cause bleeding, angiotensin converting enzyme (ACE) inhibitors such as captopril and lisinopril for high blood pressure, diuretics such as furosemide (lasix) and hydrochlorothiazide also used for high blood pressure treatment and medicines for diabetes medications as it may alter the blood sugar levels and lithium.

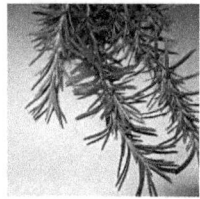

***

Sage

Sage contains vitamins A, B complex, C, E, K and the mineral calcium, copper and magnesium. It also has astringent properties which are perfect for oily skincare and hair care products. Sage has been show by some clinical trials to raise the mood and lower anxiety and it is therefore used to treat depression. It is also used to improve the memory. Sage also reduces excessive sweating and the hot flashes of menopause. It is also said to reduce the mood swings associated with menopause. It is also used to whiten teeth.

St John's Wort Flowers And Leaves

St John's Wort flowers and leaves have anti-depressant, anti-inflammatory, antiseptic properties. They are used to relieve mild depression, and manage mild eczema.

Do not use/ avoid St John's wort if you are allergic to it, have major or severe depression and bipolar disorder, are pregnant, breastfeeding or trying to get pregnant. Do not use/ avoid St John's wort if you are going to have surgery in five days, are taking digoxin for the heart, antiretroviral medicines used to treat HIV/ AIDS, if you are taking medications to treat depression as it could result in the dangerous serotonin syndrome. These antidepressant medications include serotonin reuptake inhibitors (SSRIs) such as citalopram, fluoxetine and sertraline, tricyclic antidepressants such as amitriptyline and imipramine, monoamine oxidase inhibitors (MAOIs) such as phenelzine and tranylcypromine.

***

Witch Hazel

Witch hazel is used to manage oily skin.

It is an astringent which tightens the pores and removes excessive oils. It also has healing properties.

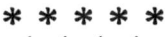

8

NATURAL PRESERVATIVES

Natural preservatives used to make skin care products include:

Rosemary Oleoresin

Rosemary oleoresin, which is also known as ROE, is a natural antioxidant extracted from the rosemary herb. It contains carnosic acid which extends the shelf life of homemade products by reducing the oxidation of their natural ingredients.

***

Vitamin E Oil

Vitamin E oil which usually comes as a mixture of tocopherols is natural antioxidant extracted from vegetable oils. Vitamin E oil is heat stable and can be used to extend the shelf life of products which do not contain water.

Grapefruit Seed Extract

Grapefruit seed extract is rich in vitamins C and E which are natural antioxidants. It is also able to kill or inhibit the growth of bacteria and fungi. It therefore functions both as a broad spectrum preservative and as an antioxidant.

###

ABOUT THE AUTHOR

Dr. Miriam Kinai is a medical doctor and a certified clinical aromatherapy practitioner.

You can visit her blog at http://www.MyBlogBookClub.com or follow her on twitter at http://twitter.com/AlmasiHealth

Email enquiries to almasihealthcare@yahoo.com with BOOKS as your subject.

HOW TO MAKE NATURAL SKIN CARE PRODUCTS SERIES

Books in this series include:

* How to Make Natural Anti-Wrinkle Creams and Anti-Aging Serums

* How to Make Natural Bath and Body Oils

* How to Make Natural Bath Bombs

* How to Make Natural Bath Cookies

* How to Make Natural Bath Melts

* How to Make Natural Bath Milks

* How to Make Natural Bath Salts

* How to Make Natural Bath Teas

* How to Make Natural Body Butters

* How to Make Natural Body Lotions

* How to Make Natural Body Scrubs

* How to Make Natural Body Wash

* How to Make Natural Cold Cream

* How to Make Natural Face Scrubs

* How to Make Natural Healing Balms

* How to Make Natural Herb Infused Oils

* How to Make Natural Massage Bars

* How to Make Natural Soap

* How to Make Natural Solid and Liquid Castile Soap

* How to Make Natural Solid and Liquid Perfumes

* How to Make Natural Sunscreen Lotions

* How to Make Natural Toothpaste, Tooth Whitening Powder and Mouthwash

* How to Make Ubtan Powder

*****

SIMPLIFIED MEDICINE

Simplified Medicine uses plain and easy to understand English to teach you about the causes, risk factors, symptoms, tests, treatment, prognosis and prevention of numerous diseases like:

* Bile Duct Cancer

* Osteosarcoma (Bone Cancer)

* Throat Cancer

* Congestive Heart Failure

* Legionnaire's Disease

* West Nile Virus

* Cryptosporidiosis

* Cyclospora

* Polymyalgia Rheumatica

* Sarcoidosis

* Alcoholic liver cirrhosis

* Dry Drowning

* Prosopagnosia

*****

HERBS AND SPICES FOR THE COOK, HEALER AND BEAUTICIAN

Herbs and Spices for the Cook, Healer and Beautician uses color pictures and clear explanations to teach you about more than 70 healing herbs and spices.

You will learn about their:

* Therapeutic (healing) uses

* Drug interactions

* Contraindications (when not to use them)

* Cooking tips

* Beauty tips

*****

MEDICAL AROMATHERAPY FOR HEALTH PROFESSIONALS

Medical Aromatherapy for Healthcare Professionals by Dr Miriam Kinai teaches you how to use essential oils to treat physical diseases and emotional disorders.

The author's experience as a medical doctor and clinical aromatherapy practitioner have enabled her to write a highly informative guide for those who want to utilize the healing benefits of these natural plant essences.

You will discover how to use essential oils to:

* Treat skin diseases like acne, eczema and psoriasis

* Treat other physical diseases like high blood pressure, arthritis, coughs and colds

* Manage mental and emotional conditions like anxiety, depression, anger and stress

* Relieve the symptoms of menopause and premenstrual tension

* Lessen insomnia and impotence

Medical Aromatherapy for Healthcare Professionals is therefore an essential resource for holistic healthcare practitioners like massage therapists, naturopaths and herbalists.

It is also a useful resource for conventional medicine healthcare providers like physicians and nurses who want to begin practicing integrative medicine and for patients who want to improve their health naturally by using aromatherapy oils.

*****

AROMATHERAPY COURSE

Aromatherapy Course by Dr Miriam Kinai tutors you on how to use essential oils to improve your physical, mental and emotional well being.

The author's experience as a medical doctor and clinical aromatherapy practitioner have enabled her to create a highly informative course on how to use these natural plant essences.

You will learn:

* The safety information and therapeutic uses of essential oils like clary sage, eucalyptus, geranium, grapefruit, lavender, lemon, lemongrass, marjoram, orange (sweet), patchouli, peppermint, Roman chamomile, rose, rosemary, sandalwood, spearmint, tea tree and ylang ylang.

* The safety information and therapeutic uses of carrier oils like apricot kernel oil, avocado oil, borage seed oil, calendula oil, carrot seed oil, castor oil, evening primrose oil, fractionated coconut oil, jojoba, olive oil, rosehip oil, sunflower oil, sweet almond oil and virgin coconut oil.

* How to blend essential oils

* How to dilute essential oils with carrier oils

* How to administer essential oils

* How to make natural healing products from numerous aromatherapy recipes

* How to utilize the healing benefits of essentials oils even if you do not have prior training in aromatherapy

The Aromatherapy Course will leave you with a clear understanding of how you can heal yourself and your family naturally by using essentials oils on your body and in your home.

*****

CHRISTIAN LIFE COACHING HANDBOOK

Christian Life Coaching Handbook offers a Biblical approach to managing different aspects of life.

You will learn:

* Christian anger management

* Christian conflict resolution

* Christian depression treatment

* Christian goal setting

* Christian marital stress management

* Christian stress management

* How to assert yourself

* How to defeat fear

* How to love yourself

* How to overcome shyness

* How to resist temptation

* How to stop being a people pleaser

*****

CHRISTIAN SPIRITUAL WARFARE

Christian Spiritual Warfare teaches you the awesome Bible verses you can use as spiritual warfare prayers, Christian affirmations and in your Christian meditation sessions as you fight your spiritual battles.

You will learn how to fight for the following with Bible verses:

* Marriage * Children * Health

* Christian Faith * Christian Ministry

* Country

* Finances * Job * Business

* Peace of Mind * Restoration * Self Esteem * Self Love

You will also learn how to fight against the following with Bible verses:

* Addiction * Temptation

* Being Single * Infertility

* Opposition * Oppression

* Worry * Fear

* Feelings of Condemnation * Confusion

* Danger * Death * Despair * Discouragement

* Impatience * Insomnia * Laziness * Loneliness

* Poverty * Pride * Sadness

* Vengeance * Weakness

* A Foul Mouth * Lying

*****

DARK SKIN DERMATOLOGY COLOR ATLAS

Dark Skin Dermatology Color Atlas is filled with clear explanations and color photos of skin, hair, and nail diseases affecting people with skin of color or Fitzpatrick skin types IV, V, and VI.

Topics covered include Acne Vulgaris, Alopecia Areata, Anal Warts, Angioedema, Aphthous Ulcers, Atopic Dermatitis, Blastomycosis, Blister Beetle Dermatitis or Nairobi Fly Dermatitis, Cellulitis, Chronic Ulcers, Confetti Hypopigmentation, Cutaneous T Cell Lymphoma, Cutaneous Tuberculosis, Dermatitis Artefacta, Erythema Nodosum,

Exfoliative Erythroderma, Gianotti Crosti Syndrome, Hand Dermatitis, Hemangioma, Herpes Zoster, Ichthyosis, Ingrown Toenails, Irritant Contact Dermatitis, Kaposi Sarcoma, Keloids, Keratoderma Blenorrhagica, Klippel Trenaunay Weber Syndrome, Leishmaniasis, Leprosy, Leukonychia, Lichen Nitidus, Lichen Planus,

Lichenoid Drug Eruption, Linear Epidermal Nevus, Linear IgA Dermatosis (LAD), Lipodermatosclerosis, Lymphangioma Circumscriptum, Miliaria, Molluscum Contagiosum, Neurofibromatosis, Nickel Dermatitis, Onychomadesis, Onychomycosis, Palmoplantar Eccrine Hidradenitis, Papular Pruritic Eruption (PPE), Paronychia, Pellagra, Pemphigus Foliaceous,

Pemphigus Vulgaris, Piebaldism, Pityriasis Rosea, Pityriasis Rubra Pilaris, Plantar Hyperkeratosis, Plantar Warts, Poikiloderma, Postinflammatory Hyperpigmentation and Hypopigmentation, Post Topical Steroids Hypopigmentation, Psoriasis, Pyogenic Granuloma or Lobular Capillary Hemangioma, Scabies, Seborrheic Dermatitis, Steven Johnson Syndrome (SJS) and Toxic Epidermal Necrolysis (TEN),

Sunburn, Systemic Sclerosis, Tinea Capitis, Tinea Pedis, Tinea Versicolor, Traction Alopecia, Urticaria, Vasculitis, Vitiligo, and Xanthelasma.

*****